WEIGHT GAIN SMOOTHIE RECIPES

Quick and Delicious Smoothies For Adding Healthy Calories To Your Diet

Corey Pearce

Copyright © 2023 Corey Pearce

GET ACCESS TO MORE BOOKS FROM THIS AUTHOR

Table of Contents

THIS PAGE WAS INTENTIONALLY LEFT BLANK

Introduction

Hey there! Let me tell you about this amazing woman who wished to add some weight. She had a lightning-fast metabolism and was often on the move, which made it impossible for her to put on any pounds. Determined to rectify that, she paid a visit to her doctor for help.

The doctor advised she try adding extra calories to her diet. Inspired by this notion, she thought, why not try preparing some great smoothies? Smoothies appeared like the ideal way to cram in more calories and minerals without feeling overloaded.

So, our woman decided to go online and look for weight gain smoothie recipes. And guess what? She discovered a book title "**Weight Gain Smoothie Recipes**" that incorporated things like peanut butter, bananas, honey, oats, protein powder, yogurt, and milk. She was absolutely thrilled to give them a whirl!

First up, she whipped up a peanut butter banana smoothie. She combined smooth peanut butter, a ripe banana, a tablespoon of honey, some ice, and milk. Let me tell you, that smoothie came out simply amazing. It left her feeling fulfilled and invigorated.

Next on the list was an oats smoothie. She blended cooked oats, a banana, a tablespoon of honey, a scoop of protein powder, and milk. Oh my, the smoothie was creamy and wonderful. She enjoyed it so much that she could have easily eaten it for breakfast every single day!

Feeling daring, she decided to try a yogurt smoothie as well. She combined plain yogurt, a banana, a tablespoon of honey, and milk. Talk about a wonderful way to start the day—it was light, creamy, and completely hit the mark.

As she began trying out various smoothie recipes, she learned how easy and fun it was to produce healthy and appetizing weight gain smoothies. The results were wonderful! She began to experiment with different variants of these dishes every week. Consistently drinking these smoothies each day started to pay off, and she began to see the results she had been striving for. She was happy to have finally discovered a technique to gain weight without losing her health.

If you're likewise trying to put on some weight without jeopardizing your well-being, don't spend any more time. Grab a copy of Weight Gain Smoothie Recipes right now! Inside this book, you'll uncover the key to healthy weight growth. The meals are tasty, healthful, and very simple to create. So why wait? Get mixing and start your weight gain adventure now!

Discover the perfect weight gain solution with our tasty smoothie recipes! Packed with calorie-dense ingredients like peanut butter, bananas, oats, and protein powder, these nutrient-rich mixes are intended to help you accomplish your weight gain objectives. Indulge in creamy, delicious smoothies that feed your body while giving the additional calories you need. Get ready to experience a delightful journey toward a healthier, fuller self. Try our Weight Gain Smoothie Recipes now and experience the pleasure of gaining weight without compromising flavor or nutrients!

THIS PAGE WAS INTENTIONALLY LEFT BLANK

Chapter 1: Understanding smoothie for weight gain

Smoothies are a terrific method to gain weight and develop muscle. Prepared with a blend of high-calorie components, such as fruits, nut butters, and protein powders, they may help you make your daily calorie target and obtain more of the nutrients you need to accomplish your weight gain and muscle development objectives.

While producing a smoothie for weight gain, it's crucial to use components that are rich in both calories and nutrients. Start with a liquid foundation, such as milk, almond milk, coconut milk, or oat milk, since they are all richer in calories than water.

Next, add protein powder, nut butters, and/or avocado for an extra boost of calories and protein. You may also add Greek yogurt for a creamy texture and an added boost of protein.

Finally, add fruits and/or vegetables for taste and additional vitamins and minerals. Bananas are a terrific alternative, since they are heavy in calories and potassium, or you may select berries, mangoes, avocados, and other fruits for a range of tastes and minerals. If you need more calories, you may add nut butters or nut-based products like coconut oil or almond butter.

Lastly, add a sweetener, such as honey, agave nectar, or stevia, to make your smoothie taste even better. You may also add spices and/or superfoods like chia seeds, flax seeds, or spirulina for an added nutritious boost.

Making a nutritious and balanced smoothie for weight gain doesn't have to be complex. With a few basic ingredients, you can produce a tasty and healthy smoothie that will help you attain your objectives.

By mixing the correct components, you may prepare a smoothie that will give you with the calories and nutrients you need to meet your weight gain and muscle development objectives. With a few easy steps, you can produce a delightful and healthy smoothie that will help you attain your objectives.

Health Benefits of smoothie for weight gain

Smoothies are a terrific strategy to gain weight and increase your general health. Not only are they wonderfully tasty, but they are also packed with nutrients and calories that will help you gain weight in a healthy manner. In this post, we'll be addressing the health advantages of smoothies for weight growth.

First of all, smoothies are highly filling and a wonderful way to get in a lot of calories fast. Since they're made up of a range of fruits and vegetables, they supply a diverse assortment of vitamins, minerals, and other critical ingredients that your body needs. Smoothies also include lots of fiber, which helps keep you feeling full and may help you avoid overeating.

In addition to supplying calories, smoothies also include lots of antioxidants, which help protect your body's cells from harm caused by free radicals. This may help decrease inflammation and enhance general health. Smoothies are also a terrific way to get in important proteins and healthy fats, which help build muscle and keep you feeling full.

Smoothies are also quite simple to create and may be swiftly made in the morning. All you need are some fresh fruit, a blender, and a beverage such as milk or water. You may also put in additional ingredients such as Greek yogurt, peanut butter, or oats to give your smoothie more texture and taste.

Lastly, smoothies are a terrific way to get in enough of calories without having to consume substantial meals throughout the day. This might be particularly advantageous if you're short on time or are attempting to gain weight in a healthy way.

Overall, smoothies are a good option for weight growth and general wellness. Not only do they supply a vast assortment of necessary nutrients, but they are also wonderfully satisfying and may be swiftly cooked. So if you're seeking to gain weight in a healthy manner, be sure to give smoothies a try.

Chapter 2: Meal Plan For Healthy Weight Gain

Day 1: Green Smoothie

INGREDIENTS:

-1 banana

-1 cup spinach

-1 cup almond milk

-1 tbsp almond butter

-1 tbsp chia seeds

INSTRUCTIONS:

-Add all ingredients to a blender.

-Blend until smooth.

-Serve immediately.

Prep Time: 5 minutes

Day 2: Apple Cinnamon Smoothie

INGREDIENTS:

-1 banana

-1 apple

-1/2 cup oats

-1 tbsp almond butter

-1 tbsp honey

-1 teaspoon cinnamon

INSTRUCTIONS:
-Add all items to a blender.
-Blend until smooth.
-Serve immediately.
Prep Time: 5 minutes

Day 3: Peanut Butter Banana Smoothie

INGREDIENTS:
-1 banana
-1 cup almond milk
-1 tablespoon honey
-1 tablespoon peanut butter
-1 teaspoon chia seeds

INSTRUCTIONS:
-Add all ingredients to a blender.
-Blend until smooth.
-Serve immediately.
Prep Time: 5 minutes

Day 4: Avocado Coconut Smoothie

INGREDIENTS:
-1 avocado
-1 cup coconut milk
-1 tbsp honey
-1 tablespoon almond butter

-1 teaspoon chia seeds

INSTRUCTIONS:
-Add all ingredients to a blender.
-Blend until smooth.
-Serve immediately.
Prep Time: 5 minutes

Day 5: Chocolate Peanut Butter Smoothie

INGREDIENTS:
-1 banana
-1 cup almond milk
-1 tbsp cocoa powder
-1 tbsp peanut butter
-1 teaspoon chia seeds

INSTRUCTIONS:
-Add all ingredients to a blender.
-Blend until smooth.
-Serve immediately.
Prep Time: 5 minutes

Day 6: Berry Coconut Smoothie

INGREDIENTS:
-1 cup mixed berries
-1 cup coconut milk

-1 tablespoon honey
-1 tablespoon almond butter
-1 teaspoon chia seeds

INSTRUCTIONS:
-Add all ingredients to a blender.
-Blend until smooth.
-Serve immediately.
Prep Time: 5 minutes

Day 7: Mango Pineapple Smoothie

INGREDIENTS:
-1 cup mango
-1 cup pineapple
-1 tablespoon honey
-1 tablespoon almond butter
-1 teaspoon chia seeds

INSTRUCTIONS:
-Add all ingredients to a blender.
-Blend until smooth.
-Serve immediately.
Prep Time: 5 minutes

Day 8: Almond Butter Banana Smoothie

INGREDIENTS:

-1 banana

-1 cup almond milk

-1 tablespoon honey

-1 tablespoon almond butter

-1 teaspoon chia seeds

INSTRUCTIONS:

-Add all ingredients to a blender.

-Blend until smooth.

-Serve immediately.

Prep Time: 5 minutes

Day 9: Peach Coconut Smoothie

INGREDIENTS:

-1 cup peaches

-1 cup coconut milk

-1 tablespoon honey

-1 tablespoon almond butter

-1 teaspoon chia seeds

INSTRUCTIONS:

-Add all ingredients to a blender.

-Blend until smooth.

-Serve immediately.

Prep Time: 5 minutes

Day 10: Hemp Seed Smoothie

INGREDIENTS:

-1 banana

-1 cup almond milk

-1 tbsp honey

-1 tablespoon hemp seeds

-1 teaspoon chia seeds

INSTRUCTIONS:

-Add all ingredients to a blender.

-Blend until smooth.

-Serve immediately.

Prep Time: 5 minutes

Day 11: Almond Milk Smoothie

INGREDIENTS:

-1 banana

-1 cup almond milk

-1 tablespoon honey

-1 tablespoon almond butter

-1 teaspoon chia seeds

INSTRUCTIONS:

-Add all ingredients to a blender.

-Blend until smooth.

-Serve immediately.
Prep Time: 5 minutes

Day 12: Peanut Butter Oat Smoothie

INGREDIENTS:

-1 banana

-1/2 cup oats

-1 tbsp honey

-1 tablespoon peanut butter

-1 teaspoon chia seeds

INSTRUCTIONS:

-Add all ingredients to a blender.

-Blend until smooth.

-Serve immediately.

Prep Time: 5 minutes

Day 13: Blueberry Coconut Smoothie

INGREDIENTS:

-1 cup blueberries

-1 cup coconut milk

-1 tablespoon honey

-1 tablespoon almond butter

-1 teaspoon chia seeds

INSTRUCTIONS:
-Add all ingredients to a blender.
-Blend until smooth.
-Serve immediately.
Prep Time: 5 minutes

Day 14: Beetroot Smoothie

INGREDIENTS:
-1 banana
-1 cup almond milk
-1/2 cup beetroot
-1 tablespoon almond butter
-1 teaspoon chia seeds

INSTRUCTIONS:
-Add all ingredients to a blender.
-Blend until smooth.
-Serve immediately.
Prep Time: 5 minutes

Day 15: Oat Almond Smoothie

INGREDIENTS:
-1 banana
-1/2 cup oats
-1 tbsp honey
-1 tablespoon almond butter
-1 teaspoon chia seeds

INSTRUCTIONS:
-Add all ingredients to a blender.
-Blend until smooth.
-Serve immediately.
Prep Time: 5 minutes

Day 16: Coconut Banana Smoothie

INGREDIENTS:
-1 banana
-1 cup coconut milk
-1 tablespoon honey
-1 tablespoon almond butter \s-1 teaspoon chia seeds

INSTRUCTIONS:
-Add all ingredients to a blender.
-Blend until smooth.
-Serve immediately.
Prep Time: 5 minutes

Day 17: Strawberry Coconut Smoothie

INGREDIENTS:
-1 cup strawberries
-1 cup coconut milk
-1 tablespoon honey

-1 tablespoon almond butter
-1 teaspoon chia seeds

INSTRUCTIONS:
-Add all ingredients to a blender.
-Blend until smooth.
-Serve immediately.
Prep Time: 5 minutes

Day 18: Cacao Coconut Smoothie

INGREDIENTS:
-1 banana
-1 cup coconut milk
-1 tablespoon honey
-1 tablespoon cacao powder
-1 teaspoon chia seeds

INSTRUCTIONS:
-Add all ingredients to a blender.
-Blend until smooth.
-Serve immediately.
Prep Time: 5 minutes

Day 19: Apple Peanut Butter Smoothie

INGREDIENTS:
-1 apple

-1 cup almond milk
-1 tablespoon honey
-1 tablespoon peanut butter
-1 teaspoon chia seeds

INSTRUCTIONS:
-Add all ingredients to a blender.
-Blend until smooth.
-Serve immediately.
Prep Time: 5 minutes

Day 20: Banana Oat Smoothie
INGREDIENTS:
-1 banana
-1/2 cup oats
-1 tbsp honeyu
-1 tablespoon almond butter
-1 teaspoon chia seeds

INSTRUCTIONS:
-Add all ingredients to a blender.
-Blend until smooth.
-Serve immediately.
Prep Time: 5 minutes

Day 21: Avocado Chocolate Smoothie

INGREDIENTS:

-1 avocado

-1 cup almond milk

-1 tablespoon honey

-1 tablespoon cocoa powder

-1 teaspoon chia seeds

INSTRUCTIONS:

-Add all ingredients to a blender.

-Blend until smooth.

-Serve immediately.

Prep Time: 5 minutes

Day 22: Mango Coconut Smoothie

INGREDIENTS:

-1 cup mango

-1 cup coconut milk

-1 tbsp honey

-1 tablespoon almond butter

-1 teaspoon chia seeds

INSTRUCTIONS:

-Add all ingredients to a blender.

-Blend until smooth.

-Serve immediately.

Prep Time: 5 minutes

Day 23: Peanut Butter Banana Smoothie

INGREDIENTS:

-1 banana

-1 cup almond milk

-1 tablespoon honey

-1 tablespoon peanut butter

-1 teaspoon chia seeds

INSTRUCTIONS:

-Add all ingredients to a blender.

-Blend until smooth.

-Serve immediately.

Prep Time: 5 minutes

Day 24: Chocolate Almond Smoothie

INGREDIENTS:

-1 banana

-1 cup almond milk

-1 tbsp cocoa powder

-1 tbsp almond butter

-1 teaspoon chia seeds

INSTRUCTIONS:

-Add all ingredients to a blender.

-Blend until smooth.
-Serve immediately.
Prep Time: 5 minutes

Day 25: Spinach Almond Smoothie

INGREDIENTS:

-1 banana
-1 cup spinach
-1 tablespoon honey
-1 tablespoon almond butter
-1 teaspoon chia seeds

INSTRUCTIONS:

-Add all ingredients to a blender.
-Blend until smooth.
-Serve immediately.
Prep Time: 5 minutes

Day 26: Berry Hemp Smoothie

INGREDIENTS:

-1 cup mixed berries
-1 cup almond milk
-1 tablespoon honey
-1 tablespoon hemp seeds
-1 teaspoon chia seeds

INSTRUCTIONS:

-Add all ingredients to a blender.

-Blend until smooth.

-Serve immediately.

Prep Time: 5 minutes

Day 27: Pineapple Coconut Smoothie

INGREDIENTS:

-1 cup pineapple

-1 cup coconut milk

-1 tbsp honey

-1 tablespoon almond butter

-1 teaspoon chia seeds

INSTRUCTIONS:

-Add all ingredients to a blender.

-Blend until smooth.

-Serve immediately.

Prep Time: 5 minutes

Day 28: Beetroot Oat Smoothie

INGREDIENTS:

-1/2 cup beets

-1/2 cup oats

-1 tbsp honey

-1 tablespoon almond butter

-1 teaspoon chia seeds

INSTRUCTIONS:
-Add all items to a blender.
-Blend until smooth.
-Serve immediately.
Prep Time: 5 minutes

Day 29: Apple Cinnamon Smoothie

INGREDIENTS:
-1 apple
-1 cup almond milk
-1 tablespoon honey
-1 tablespoon almond butter
-1 teaspoon cinnamon

INSTRUCTIONS:
-Add all ingredients to a blender.
-Blend until smooth.
-Serve immediately.
Prep Time: 5 minutes

Day 30: Blueberry Almond Smoothie

INGREDIENTS:
-1 cup blueberries
-1 cup almond milk

-1 tablespoon honey
-1 tablespoon almond butter
-1 teaspoon chia seeds

INSTRUCTIONS:
-Add all ingredients to a blender.
-Blend until smooth.
-Serve immediately.
Prep Time: 5 minutes

THIS PAGE WAS INTENTIONALLY LEFT BLANK

Chapter 3: Banana Protein Smoothie

Strawberry Banana Protein Smoothie

INTRODUCTION:
This smoothie is a delicious and nutritious way to start your day. It's packed with protein and sweetened with strawberries, so it's sure to keep you full and energized.

INGREDIENTS:
-1 ripe banana
-1 cup frozen strawberries
-1 scoop vanilla protein powder
-1 cup almond milk
-1 tablespoon honey
-1 teaspoon chia seeds

PREPARATION METHOD:
-Add the banana, strawberries, protein powder, almond milk, honey, and chia seeds to a blender.
-Blend until smooth and creamy.
-Pour into a glass and enjoy.

Prep Time: 5 minutes

Peanut Butter Banana Protein Smoothie

INTRODUCTION:
This smoothie is a creamy and tasty way to get your daily dose of protein. It's made with banana, peanut butter, and protein powder, so it's sure to give you the energy you need.

INGREDIENTS:
-1 ripe banana
-1 tablespoon peanut butter
-1 scoop vanilla protein powder
-1 cup almond milk
-1 tablespoon honey
-1 teaspoon chia seeds

PREPARATION METHOD:
-Add the banana, peanut butter, protein powder, almond milk, honey, and chia seeds to a blender.
-Blend until smooth and creamy.
-Pour into a glass and enjoy.

Prep Time: 5 minutes

Chocolate Banana Protein Smoothie:

INTRODUCTION:
This smoothie is a decadent and nutritious way to get your daily dose of protein. It's made with banana, cocoa powder, and protein powder, so it's sure to give you the energy you need.

INGREDIENTS:
-1 ripe banana

-2 tablespoons cocoa powder

-1 scoop chocolate protein powder

-1 cup almond milk

-1 tablespoon honey

-1 teaspoon chia seeds

PREPARATION METHOD:
-Add the banana, cocoa powder, protein powder, almond milk, honey, and chia seeds to a blender.

-Blend until smooth and creamy.

-Pour into a glass and enjoy.

Prep Time: 5 minutes

Blueberry Banana Protein Smoothie

INTRODUCTION:

This smoothie is a fruity and nutritious way to get your daily dose of protein. It's made with banana, blueberries, and protein powder, so it's sure to give you the energy you need.

INGREDIENTS:

-1 ripe banana
-1 cup frozen blueberries
-1 scoop vanilla protein powder
-1 cup almond milk
-1 tablespoon honey
-1 teaspoon chia seeds

PREPARATION METHOD:

-Add the banana, blueberries, protein powder, almond milk, honey, and chia seeds to a blender.
-Blend until smooth and creamy.
-Pour into a glass and enjoy.

Prep Time: 5 minutes

Coconut Banana Protein Smoothie

INTRODUCTION:

This smoothie is a creamy and delicious way to get your daily dose of protein. It's made with banana, coconut, and protein powder, so it's sure to give you the energy you need.

INGREDIENTS:

-1 ripe banana

-1 tablespoon shredded coconut

-1 scoop vanilla protein powder

-1 cup almond milk

-1 tablespoon honey

-1 teaspoon chia seeds

PREPARATION METHOD:

-Add the banana, coconut, protein powder, almond milk, honey, and chia seeds to a blender.

-Blend until smooth and creamy.

-Pour into a glass and enjoy.

Prep Time: 5 minutes

THIS PAGE WAS INTENTIONALLY LEFT BLANK

Chapter 4: Peanut Butter Oatmeal Smoothie

Chocolate Peanut Butter Oatmeal Smoothie

INTRODUCTION:
This smoothie is a delicious combination of chocolate and peanut butter flavors, with a hint of oatmeal for added texture.

INGREDIENTS:
- ½ cup of oats
- 1 banana
- 2 tablespoons of cocoa powder
- 2 tablespoons of peanut butter
- 1 teaspoon of vanilla extract
- 1 cup of milk
- 1 teaspoon of honey and ice cubes.

PREPARATION METHOD:
- In a blender, combine all of the ingredients and mix until smooth.
- Blend in the ice cubes until the desired consistency is reached.

Prep Time: 5 minutes

Banana Peanut Butter Oatmeal Smoothie

INTRODUCTION:
This smoothie is a creamy and healthy treat, perfect for breakfast or a snack. It's packed with protein and fiber to keep you full and energized all day.

INGREDIENTS:
- ½ cup of oats
- 1 banana
- 2 tablespoons of peanut butter
- 1 teaspoon of vanilla extract
- 1 cup of milk, 1 teaspoon of honey and ice cubes.

PREPARATION METHOD:
- In a blender, combine all of the ingredients and mix until smooth
- Blend in the ice cubes until the desired consistency is reached.
Prep Time: 5 minutes

Caramel Peanut Butter Oatmeal Smoothie

INTRODUCTION:

This smoothie is a delicious mix of sweet and salty flavors, perfect for a quick and easy breakfast or snack.

INGREDIENTS:

- ½ cup of oats
- 1 banana
- 2 tablespoons of caramel sauce
- 2 tablespoons of peanut butter
- 1 teaspoon of vanilla extract
- 1 cup of milk
- 1 teaspoon of honey and ice cubes.

PREPARATION METHOD:

- In a blender, combine all of the ingredients and mix until smooth
- Blend in the ice cubes until the desired consistency is reached.

Prep Time: 5 minutes

Strawberry ´ Peanut Butter Oatmeal Smoothie

INTRODUCTION:
This smoothie is a perfect combination of sweet and tart flavors. The strawberries and peanut butter provide a delicious and creamy texture.

INGREDIENTS:
- ½ cup of oats
- 1 banana
- ½ cup of chopped fresh strawberries
- 2 tablespoons of peanut butter
- 1 teaspoon of vanilla extract
- 1 cup of milk
- 1 teaspoon of honey and ice cubes.

PREPARATION METHOD:
- In a blender, combine all of the ingredients and mix until smooth
- Blend in the ice cubes until the desired consistency is reached.
Prep Time: 5 minutes

Blueberry Peanut Butter Oatmeal Smoothie

INTRODUCTION:

This smoothie is a healthy and delicious blend of sweet and tart flavors. The blueberries and peanut butter provide a great flavor combination that's sure to please.

INGREDIENTS:

- ½ cup of oats
- 1 banana
- ½ cup of fresh blueberries
- 2 tablespoons of peanut butter
- 1 teaspoon of vanilla extract
- 1 cup of milk, 1 teaspoon of honey and ice cubes.

PREPARATION METHOD:

- In a blender, combine all of the ingredients and mix until smooth
- Blend in the ice cubes until the desired consistency is reached.
Prep Time: 5 minutes

THIS PAGE WAS INTENTIONALLY LEFT BLANK

Chapter 6: Chocolate Coconut Protein Smoothie

Choco Coconut Banana Protein Smoothie

INTRODUCTION:
This smoothie is a great way to start your day with a delicious blend of sweet flavors. It's packed with protein, healthy fats and natural sweetness for a powerful morning boost.

INGREDIENTS:
- 1 banana
- 1 scoop of chocolate protein powder
- 1 cup of unsweetened almond milk
- 1/2 cup of coconut flakes
- 1 teaspoon of honey
- 1 tablespoon of cocoa powder

PREPARATION METHOD:
1. Place banana, protein powder, almond milk, coconut flakes, honey and cocoa powder in a blender.
2. Blend until smooth.
3. Pour into a glass and enjoy!

Prep Time: 5 minutes

Choco Coconut Peanut Butter Protein Smoothie

INTRODUCTION:
This smoothie is a delicious and filling way to get your daily protein and energy boost. It's packed with creamy peanut butter, rich cocoa, and sweet coconut flavors.

INGREDIENTS:
- 1 banana
- 1 scoop of chocolate protein powder
- 1 cup of unsweetened almond milk
- 1/2 cup of coconut flakes
- 1 tablespoon of peanut butter
- 1 tablespoon of cocoa powder

PREPARATION METHOD:
1. Place banana, protein powder, almond milk, coconut flakes, peanut butter and cocoa powder in a blender.
2. Blend until smooth.
3. Pour into a glass and enjoy!

Prep Time: 5 minutes

Choco Coconut Avocado Protein Smoothie

INTRODUCTION:

This smoothie is a creamy, nutrient-packed way to get your daily protein and energy boost. It's packed with healthy fats, creamy avocado, and sweet coconut flavors.

INGREDIENTS:

- 1 banana
- 1 scoop of chocolate protein powder
- 1 cup of unsweetened almond milk
- 1/2 cup of coconut flakes
- 1/4 of an avocado
- 1 tablespoon of cocoa powder

PREPARATION METHOD:

1. Place banana, protein powder, almond milk, coconut flakes, avocado and cocoa powder in a blender.
2. Blend until smooth.
3. Pour into a glass and enjoy!

Prep Time: 5 minutes

Choco Coconut Date Protein Smoothie

INTRODUCTION:
This smoothie is an indulgent yet healthy way to get your daily protein and energy boost. It's packed with natural sweetness from dates, creamy avocado, and sweet coconut flavors.

INGREDIENTS:
- 1 banana
- 1 scoop of chocolate protein powder
- 1 cup of unsweetened almond milk
- 1/2 cup of coconut flakes
- 2 dates
- 1 tablespoon of cocoa powder

PREPARATION METHOD:
1. Place banana, protein powder, almond milk, coconut flakes, dates and cocoa powder in a blender.
2. Blend until smooth.
3. Pour into a glass and enjoy!

Prep Time: 5 minutes

Choco Coconut Oat Protein Smoothie

INTRODUCTION:

This smoothie is a filling and delicious way to get your daily protein and energy boost. It's packed with creamy oats, rich cocoa, and sweet coconut flavors.

INGREDIENTS:

- 1 banana
- 1 scoop of chocolate protein powder
- 1 cup of unsweetened almond milk
- 1/2 cup of coconut flakes
- 1/4 cup of rolled oats
- 1 tablespoon of cocoa powder

PREPARATION METHOD:

1. Place banana, protein powder, almond milk, coconut flakes, oats and cocoa powder in a blender.
2. Blend until smooth.
3. Pour into a glass and enjoy!

Prep Time: 5 minutes

THIS PAGE WAS INTENTIONALLY LEFT BLANK

Chapter 6: Avocado Spinach Smoothie

Avocado Spinach Smoothie with Pineapple

INTRODUCTION:

This healthy and delicious smoothie is packed with nutrients from the spinach, avocado, and pineapple. It's a great way to start the day and keep you energized.

INGREDIENTS:

- ½ avocado
- 1 cup spinach
- 1 cup pineapple
- 1 cup almond milk
- 1 teaspoon honey
- 1 teaspoon chia seeds
- 1 teaspoon hemp hearts
- Ice

PREPARATION METHOD:

1. Add avocado, spinach, pineapple, almond milk, honey, chia seeds and hemp hearts to a blender and blend until smooth.
2. Serve over ice.

Prep Time: 10 minutes

Avocado Spinach Smoothie with Banana

INTRODUCTION:
This smoothie is a great way to get your greens while getting an extra boost of energy from the banana. It's creamy and delicious, and perfect for a mid-day snack.

INGREDIENTS:
- ½ avocado
- 1 cup spinach
- 1 banana
- 1 cup almond milk
- 1 teaspoon honey
- 1 teaspoon chia seeds
- 1 teaspoon hemp hearts
- Ice

PREPARATION METHOD:
1. Add avocado, spinach, banana, almond milk, honey, chia seeds and hemp hearts to a blender and blend until smooth.
2. Serve over ice.

Prep Time: 10 minutes

Avocado Spinach Smoothie with Coconut Milk

INTRODUCTION:

This creamy and delicious smoothie is a great way to get your greens while getting an extra boost of energy from the coconut milk. It's an excellent way to start the day.

INGREDIENTS:

- ½ avocado
- 1 cup spinach
- 1 cup coconut milk
- 1 teaspoon honey
- 1 teaspoon chia seeds
- 1 teaspoon hemp hearts
- Ice

PREPARATION METHOD:

1. Add avocado, spinach, coconut milk, honey, chia seeds and hemp hearts to a blender and blend until smooth.
2. Serve over ice.

Prep Time: 10 minutes

Avocado Spinach Smoothie with Mango

INTRODUCTION:
This smoothie is a great way to get your greens while getting an extra boost of sweetness from the mango. It's an excellent way to start the day.

INGREDIENTS:
- ½ avocado
- 1 cup spinach
- 1 cup mango
- 1 cup almond milk
- 1 teaspoon honey
- 1 teaspoon chia seeds
- 1 teaspoon hemp hearts
- Ice

PREPARATION METHOD:
1. Add avocado, spinach, mango, almond milk, honey, chia seeds and hemp hearts to a blender and blend until smooth.
2. Serve over ice.

Prep Time: 10 minutes

Avocado Spinach Smoothie with Orange

INTRODUCTION:

This smoothie is a great way to get your greens while getting an extra boost of Vitamin C from the orange. It's an excellent way to start the day.

INGREDIENTS:

- ½ avocado
- 1 cup spinach
- 1 orange
- 1 cup almond milk
- 1 teaspoon honey
- 1 teaspoon chia seeds
- 1 teaspoon hemp hearts
- Ice

PREPARATION METHOD:

1. Add avocado, spinach, orange, almond milk, honey, chia seeds and hemp hearts to a blender and blend until smooth.
2. Serve over ice.

Prep Time: 10 minutes

THIS PAGE WAS INTENTIONALLY LEFT BLANK

Chapter 7: Mango Coconut Smoothie

Mango Coconut Smoothie

INTRODUCTION:
A delicious and refreshing combination of mango and coconut creates a perfect smoothie for a summer day.

INGREDIENTS:
- 1 ripe mango, peeled and diced
- 1 cup coconut milk
- 2 tablespoons honey
- 2 tablespoons chia seeds
- 1/2 teaspoon ground ginger
- 1/2 teaspoon vanilla extract
- 2 cups ice cubes

PREPARATION METHOD:
1. In a blender, combine the mango, coconut milk, honey, chia seeds, ground ginger and vanilla extract.
2. Blend until smooth.
3. Add the ice cubes and mix until creamy.

Prep Time: 5 minutes

Tropical Mango Coconut Smoothie

INTRODUCTION:
Enjoy a taste of the tropics with this mango coconut smoothie. It's creamy, sweet and packed with tropical flavors.

INGREDIENTS:
- 1 ripe mango, peeled and diced
- 1/2 cup coconut milk
- 1/4 cup pineapple juice
- 2 tablespoons honey
- 1/2 teaspoon ground ginger
- 1/2 teaspoon ground cinnamon
- 2 cups ice cubes

PREPARATION METHOD:
1. In a blender, combine the mango, coconut milk, pineapple juice, honey, ground ginger and ground cinnamon.
2. Blend until smooth.
3. Add the ice cubes and mix until creamy.

Prep Time: 5 minutes

Mango Coconut Protein Smoothie

INTRODUCTION:

Start your day off right with this protein-packed mango coconut smoothie. It's creamy, sweet and full of plant-based protein.

INGREDIENTS:
- 1 ripe mango, peeled and diced
- 1 cup coconut milk
- 2 tablespoons honey
- 1 scoop plant-based protein powder
- 2 tablespoons chia seeds
- 1/2 teaspoon ground ginger
- 1/2 teaspoon vanilla extract
- 2 cups ice cubes

PREPARATION METHOD:

1. In a blender, combine the mango, coconut milk, honey, protein powder, chia seeds, ground ginger and vanilla extract.
2. Blend until smooth.
3. Add the ice cubes and mix until creamy.

Prep Time: 5 minutes

Mango Coconut Kefir Smoothie

INTRODUCTION:

This mango coconut kefir smoothie is a great way to get probiotics into your diet. It's creamy, sweet and full of probiotic-rich kefir.

INGREDIENTS:

- 1 ripe mango, peeled and diced
- 1 cup coconut milk
- 2 tablespoons honey
- 1 cup plain kefir
- 2 tablespoons chia seeds
- 1/2 teaspoon ground ginger
- 1/2 teaspoon vanilla extract
- 2 cups ice cubes

PREPARATION METHOD:

1. In a blender, combine the mango, coconut milk, honey, kefir, chia seeds, ground ginger and vanilla extract.
2. Blend until smooth.
3. Add the ice cubes and mix until creamy.

Prep Time: 5 minutes

Mango Coconut Green Smoothie

INTRODUCTION:

Get your daily greens in with this mango coconut green smoothie. It's creamy, sweet and full of nutritious greens.

INGREDIENTS:

- 1 ripe mango, peeled and diced
- 1 cup coconut milk
- 2 tablespoons honey
- 1 cup baby spinach
- 2 tablespoons chia seeds
- 1/2 teaspoon ground ginger
- 1/2 teaspoon vanilla extract
- 2 cups ice cubes

PREPARATION METHOD:

1. In a blender, combine the mango, coconut milk, honey, baby spinach, chia seeds, ground ginger and vanilla extract.
2. Blend until smooth.
3. Add the ice cubes and mix until creamy.

Prep Time: 5 minutes

Chapter 8: Strawberry Almond Smoothie

Strawberry Smoothie   Almond

INTRODUCTION:
This smoothie is a delicious and nutritious way to start your day! A blend of sweet strawberries, creamy almond milk, and crunchy almonds, it's a great way to get your daily dose of vitamin C and protein.

INGREDIENTS:
- 1 cup frozen strawberries
- 1 cup almond milk
- 1 tablespoon honey
- ¼ cup almonds, chopped
- Ice cubes

PREPARATION METHOD:
1. In a blender, add the frozen strawberries, almond milk, honey and almonds.
2. Blend until smooth.
3. Add in the ice cubes and blend until desired consistency is reached.
4. Serve immediately.

Prep Time: 5 minutes

Creamy Strawberry Almond Smoothie

INTRODUCTION:
This creamy strawberry almond smoothie is a delicious and healthy way to start your day! It's made with creamy almond milk, sweet strawberries, and crunchy almonds, making it a great source of vitamins and protein.

INGREDIENTS:
- 1 cup frozen strawberries
- 1 cup almond milk
- 1 tablespoon honey
- 2 tablespoons cream cheese
- ¼ cup almonds, chopped
- Ice cubes

PREPARATION METHOD:
1. In a blender, add the frozen strawberries, almond milk, honey, cream cheese, and almonds.
2. Blend until smooth.
3. Add in the ice cubes and blend until desired consistency is reached.
4. Serve immediately.

Strawberry Almond Milkshake

Prep Time: 5 minutes

INTRODUCTION:

This strawberry almond milkshake is a delicious and creamy treat! Made with sweet strawberries, creamy almond milk, and crunchy almonds, it's a great way to get your daily dose of vitamin C and protein.

INGREDIENTS:
- 1 cup frozen strawberries
- 1 cup almond milk
- ¼ cup sugar
- 2 tablespoons cream
- ¼ cup almonds, chopped
- Ice cubes

PREPARATION METHOD:

1. In a blender, add the frozen strawberries, almond milk, sugar, cream, and almonds.
2. Blend until smooth.
3. Add in the ice cubes and blend until desired consistency is reached.
4. Serve immediately.

Prep Time: 5 minutes

Strawberry Almond Protein Smoothie

INTRODUCTION:
This strawberry almond protein smoothie is a delicious and nutritious way to start your day! Made with sweet strawberries, creamy almond milk, and crunchy almonds, it's a great source of vitamins and protein.

INGREDIENTS:
• 1 cup frozen strawberries
• 1 cup almond milk
• 1 scoop protein powder
• ¼ cup almonds, chopped
• Ice cubes

PREPARATION METHOD:
1. In a blender, add the frozen strawberries, almond milk, protein powder, and almonds.
2. Blend until smooth.
3. Add in the ice cubes and blend until desired consistency is reached.
4. Serve immediately.

Prep Time: 5 minutes

Banana Strawberry Almond Smoothie

INTRODUCTION:

This banana strawberry almond smoothie is a delicious and healthy way to start your day! A blend of sweet strawberries, creamy almond milk, and crunchy almonds, it's a great way to get your daily dose of vitamin C and potassium.

INGREDIENTS:

- ½ banana, sliced
- 1 cup frozen strawberries
- 1 cup almond milk
- ¼ cup almonds, chopped
- Ice cubes

PREPARATION METHOD:

1. In a blender, add the banana, frozen strawberries, almond milk, and almonds.
2. Blend until smooth.
3. Add in the ice cubes and blend until desired consistency is reached.
4. Serve immediately.

Prep Time: 5 minutes

THIS PAGE WAS INTENTIONALLY LEFT BLANK

Chapter 9: Blueberry Oat Smoothie

Blueberry Banana Oat Smoothie

INTRODUCTION:

This blueberry banana oat smoothie is a delicious and healthy way to start your day. It is packed with antioxidants from the blueberries and fiber from the oats. The banana and almond milk add sweetness to the smoothie, making it an ideal breakfast or snack.

INGREDIENTS:

- 1/2 cup blueberries
- 1 banana
- 1/2 cup oats
- 1 cup almond milk
- 1 tablespoon honey

PREPARATION METHOD:

1. Place the oats, blueberries, banana, almond milk and honey in a blender and blend until smooth.

2. Pour the smoothie into a glass and serve immediately.

Prep time: 5 minutes

Blueberry Oat and Flax Smoothie

INTRODUCTION:
This blueberry oat and flax smoothie is a nutritious and refreshing way to start your day. The oats and flax provide healthy fiber, and the blueberries give it a delicious sweet and tart flavor.

INGREDIENTS:
- 1/2 cup blueberries
- 1 banana
- 1/2 cup oats
- 1 tablespoon flax seeds
- 1 cup almond milk
- 1 tablespoon honey

PREPARATION METHOD:
1. Place the oats, blueberries, banana, flax seeds, almond milk and honey in a blender and blend until smooth.
2. Pour the smoothie into a glass and serve immediately.

Prep time: 5 minutes

Blueberry Almond Oat Smoothie

INTRODUCTION:
This blueberry almond oat smoothie is a creamy and delicious way to start your day. The oats and almond milk provide healthy fiber, and the blueberries add a sweet and tart flavor.

INGREDIENTS:
- 1/2 cup blueberries
- 1 banana
- 1/2 cup oats
- 1 cup almond milk
- 1 tablespoon almond butter
- 1 tablespoon honey

PREPARATION METHOD:
1. Place the oats, blueberries, banana, almond milk, almond butter and honey in a blender and blend until smooth.
2. Pour the smoothie into a glass and serve immediately.

Prep time: 5 minutes

Blueberry Coconut Oat Smoothie

INTRODUCTION:
This blueberry coconut oat smoothie is a creamy and tropical treat for any time of day. The oats and coconut milk provide healthy fiber, and the blueberries add a sweet and tart flavor.

INGREDIENTS:
- 1/2 cup blueberries
- 1 banana
- 1/2 cup oats
- 1 cup coconut milk
- 1 tablespoon shredded coconut
- 1 tablespoon honey

PREPARATION METHOD:
1. Place the oats, blueberries, banana, coconut milk, shredded coconut and honey in a blender and blend until smooth.
2. Pour the smoothie into a glass and serve immediately.

Prep time: 5 minutes

Blueberry Acai Oat Smoothie

INTRODUCTION:

This blueberry acai oat smoothie is a refreshing and nutritious way to start your day. The oats and acai berries provide healthy fiber, and the blueberries add a sweet and tart flavor.

INGREDIENTS:

- 1/2 cup blueberries
- 1 banana
- 1/2 cup oats
- 1/2 cup acai berries
- 1 cup almond milk
- 1 tablespoon honey

PREPARATION METHOD:

1. Place the oats, blueberries, banana, acai berries, almond milk and honey in a blender and blend until smooth.

2. Pour the smoothie into a glass and serve immediately.

Prep time: 5 minutes

THIS PAGE WAS INTENTIONALLY LEFT BLANK

Chapter 10: Green Monster Smoothie

Berry & Coconut Green Monster Smoothie

INTRODUCTION:

Here is a delicious green monster smoothie that is full of flavor and nutrition. Berries and coconut add a tropical flavor that will make your taste buds dance.

INGREDIENTS:

-1 cup frozen berries (strawberries, raspberries or blueberries)
-1 banana
-3/4 cup coconut milk
-1/4 cup fresh spinach
-1 teaspoon honey
-1 teaspoon chia seeds

PREPARATION METHOD:

1. Blend all of the ingredients in a blender until smooth.
2. Pour into a glass and enjoy!

Prep Time: 5 minutes

Citrus & Avocado Green Monster Smoothie

INTRODUCTION:

This green monster smoothie is a great way to start your day. It is super refreshing and packed with healthy fats that will give you an energy boost.

INGREDIENTS:

-1/2 cup orange juice
-1/2 cup pineapple juice
-1 banana
-1/2 avocado
-1/4 cup fresh spinach
-1 teaspoon honey
-1 teaspoon chia seeds

PREPARATION METHOD:

1. Blend all of the ingredients in a blender until smooth..
2. Pour into a glass and enjoy!

Prep Time: 5 minutes

Mango & Ginger Green Monster Smoothie

INTRODUCTION:

This green monster smoothie is a great way to get your day started. The mango and ginger add a unique and delicious flavor that will make your taste buds sing.

INGREDIENTS:

-1 cup frozen mango

-1 banana

-3/4 cup almond milk

-1/4 cup fresh spinach

-1 teaspoon honey

-1 teaspoon fresh ginger

-1 teaspoon chia seeds

PREPARATION METHOD:

1. Blend all of the ingredients in a blender until smooth.
2. Pour into a glass and enjoy!

Prep Time: 5 minutes

Pineapple & Coconut Green Monster Smoothie

INTRODUCTION:

This green monster smoothie is a great way to get your day started. Pineapple and coconut blend together to create a tropical flavor that will take you away.

INGREDIENTS:

-1 cup frozen pineapple
-1 banana
-3/4 cup coconut milk
-1/4 cup fresh spinach
-1 teaspoon honey
-1 teaspoon chia seeds

PREPARATION METHOD:

1. Blend all of the ingredients in a blender until smooth.
2. Pour into a glass and enjoy!

Prep Time: 5 minutes

Banana & Peanut Butter Green Monster Smoothie

INTRODUCTION:

This green monster smoothie is healthy, creamy and delicious. The combination of banana and peanut butter adds a sweet and nutty flavor that is sure to please.

INGREDIENTS:

-1 banana
-1/4 cup peanut butter
-3/4 cup almond milk
-1/4 cup fresh spinach
-1 teaspoon honey
-1 teaspoon chia seeds

PREPARATION METHOD:

1. Blend all of the ingredients in a blender until smooth.
2. Pour into a glass and enjoy!

Prep Time: 5 minutes

THIS PAGE WAS INTENTIONALLY LEFT BLANK

79

Conclusion

Overall, this book has been an invaluable resource for anyone looking to gain weight in a healthy and balanced way. It contains a variety of delicious smoothie recipes that are easy to make and can be customized to fit any dietary needs.

The recipes in this book provide plenty of essential nutrients to help you reach your weight gain goals. Additionally, the book includes valuable information about the importance of nutrition and provides helpful tips to ensure that you are getting the most out of your smoothies.

The recipes in this book have been specifically designed to help you gain weight in a healthy and sustainable way, and they are sure to be a hit with anyone looking to up their calorie intake in a delicious way. With this book, you can rest assured that you will be able to create nutritious and delicious smoothies that will help you reach your weight gain goals in no time.

If truly you are looking to put on some weight in the healthiest and most delicious way possible, this book of weight gain smoothie recipes is the perfect resource for you. With its wide variety of recipes, helpful tips and essential nutritional information, this book is sure to help you reach your weight gain goals in no time.

So grab your blender, pick up this book and get ready to enjoy some delicious smoothies and a healthier you.

Contact Us

Dear valued reader,

First and foremost, I would like to express my sincere gratitude for choosing my book WEIGHT GAIN SMOOTHIE RECIPES as your guide. I hope that you found the content helpful, informative, and enjoyable to read.

As a valued customer, I would like to offer you an exclusive bonus - a free WEEKLY MEAL JOURNAL but it is attached to the paperback version.

I also want to remind you that your review/feedback is important to me. I would love to hear your thoughts, observations, questions and suggestions about the book, so that I can continue to improve and provide you with even more valuable content in the future.

You can contact me through this email: Coreyhelpdesk@gmail.com

Thank you once again for choosing my book, and I look forward to hearing from you soon!

Best regards,

Corey Pearce

Bonus - Special Meal Tracker

WEEKLY MEAL JOURNAL

DATE:...............................

MONDAY	BREAKFAST	
	LUNCH	
	DINNER	
TUESDAY	BREAKFAST	
	LUNCH	
	DINNER	
WEDNESDAY	BREAKFAST	
	LUNCH	
	DINNER	
THURSDAY	BREAKFAST	
	LUNCH	
	DINNER	
FRIDAY	BREAKFAST	
	LUNCH	
	DINNER	
SATURDAY	BREAKFAST	
	LUNCH	
	DINNER	
SUNDAY	BREAKFAST	
	LUNCH	
	DINNER	

SNACKS

NOTE

WEEKLY MEAL JOURNAL

DATE:..............................

MONDAY	BREAKFAST	
	LUNCH	
	DINNER	
TUESDAY	BREAKFAST	
	LUNCH	
	DINNER	
WEDNESDAY	BREAKFAST	
	LUNCH	
	DINNER	
THURSDAY	BREAKFAST	
	LUNCH	
	DINNER	
FRIDAY	BREAKFAST	
	LUNCH	
	DINNER	
SATURDAY	BREAKFAST	
	LUNCH	
	DINNER	
SUNDAY	BREAKFAST	
	LUNCH	
	DINNER	

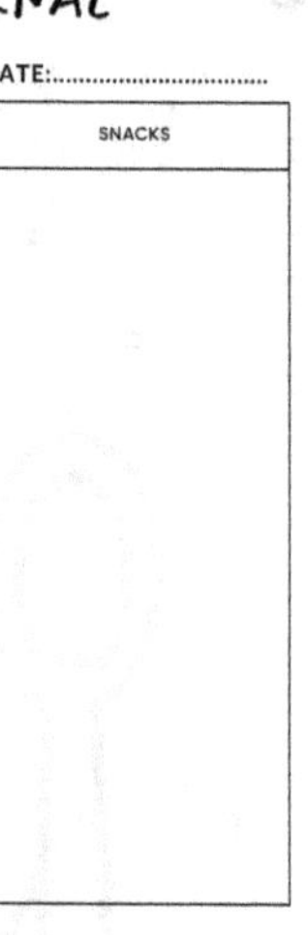

SNACKS

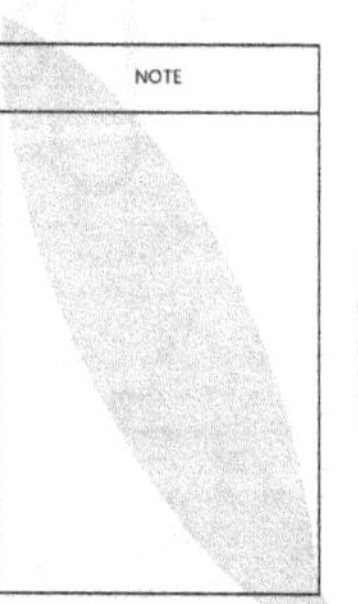

NOTE

WEEKLY MEAL JOURNAL

DATE:.................................

		MONDAY
	BREAKFAST	
MONDAY	LUNCH	
	DINNER	
	BREAKFAST	
TUESDAY	LUNCH	
	DINNER	
	BREAKFAST	
WEDNESDAY	LUNCH	
	DINNER	
	BREAKFAST	
THURSDAY	LUNCH	
	DINNER	
	BREAKFAST	
FRIDAY	LUNCH	
	DINNER	
	BREAKFAST	
SATURDAY	LUNCH	
	DINNER	
	BREAKFAST	
SUNDAY	LUNCH	
	DINNER	

SNACKS

NOTE

WEEKLY MEAL JOURNAL

DATE:..................................

MONDAY	BREAKFAST	
	LUNCH	
	DINNER	
TUESDAY	BREAKFAST	
	LUNCH	
	DINNER	
WEDNESDAY	BREAKFAST	
	LUNCH	
	DINNER	
THURSDAY	BREAKFAST	
	LUNCH	
	DINNER	
FRIDAY	BREAKFAST	
	LUNCH	
	DINNER	
SATURDAY	BREAKFAST	
	LUNCH	
	DINNER	
SUNDAY	BREAKFAST	
	LUNCH	
	DINNER	

SNACKS

NOTE

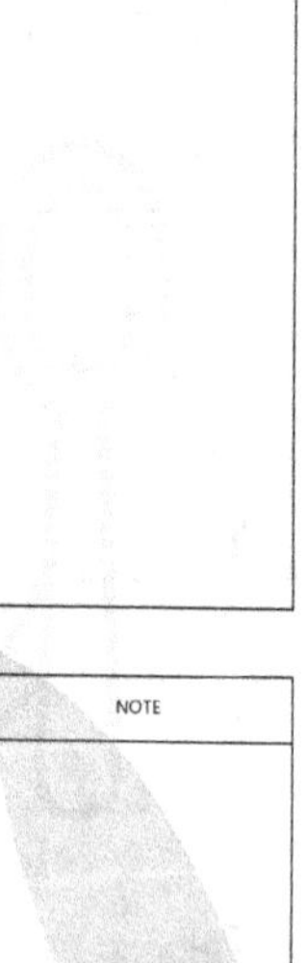

WEEKLY MEAL JOURNAL

DATE:................................

MONDAY	BREAKFAST	
	LUNCH	
	DINNER	
TUESDAY	BREAKFAST	
	LUNCH	
	DINNER	
WEDNESDAY	BREAKFAST	
	LUNCH	
	DINNER	
THURSDAY	BREAKFAST	
	LUNCH	
	DINNER	
FRIDAY	BREAKFAST	
	LUNCH	
	DINNER	
SATURDAY	BREAKFAST	
	LUNCH	
	DINNER	
SUNDAY	BREAKFAST	
	LUNCH	
	DINNER	

SNACKS

NOTE

WEEKLY MEAL JOURNAL

DATE:...................................

MONDAY	BREAKFAST	
	LUNCH	
	DINNER	
TUESDAY	BREAKFAST	
	LUNCH	
	DINNER	
WEDNESDAY	BREAKFAST	
	LUNCH	
	DINNER	
THURSDAY	BREAKFAST	
	LUNCH	
	DINNER	
FRIDAY	BREAKFAST	
	LUNCH	
	DINNER	
SATURDAY	BREAKFAST	
	LUNCH	
	DINNER	
SUNDAY	BREAKFAST	
	LUNCH	
	DINNER	

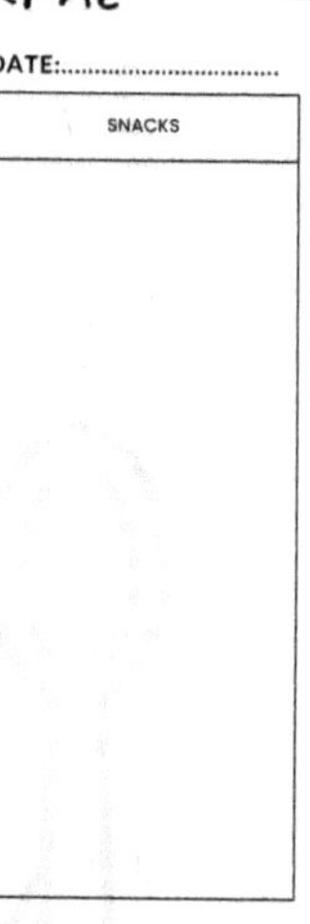

SNACKS

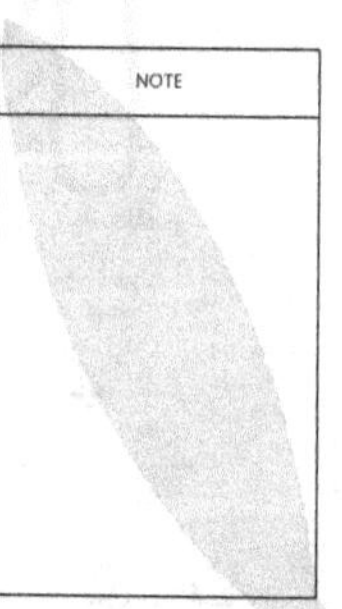

NOTE

WEEKLY MEAL JOURNAL

DATE:................................

MONDAY	BREAKFAST	
	LUNCH	
	DINNER	
TUESDAY	BREAKFAST	
	LUNCH	
	DINNER	
WEDNESDAY	BREAKFAST	
	LUNCH	
	DINNER	
THURSDAY	BREAKFAST	
	LUNCH	
	DINNER	
FRIDAY	BREAKFAST	
	LUNCH	
	DINNER	
SATURDAY	BREAKFAST	
	LUNCH	
	DINNER	
SUNDAY	BREAKFAST	
	LUNCH	
	DINNER	

SNACKS

NOTE

WEEKLY MEAL JOURNAL

DATE:...............................

MONDAY	BREAKFAST	
	LUNCH	
	DINNER	
TUESDAY	BREAKFAST	
	LUNCH	
	DINNER	
WEDNESDAY	BREAKFAST	
	LUNCH	
	DINNER	
THURSDAY	BREAKFAST	
	LUNCH	
	DINNER	
FRIDAY	BREAKFAST	
	LUNCH	
	DINNER	
SATURDAY	BREAKFAST	
	LUNCH	
	DINNER	
SUNDAY	BREAKFAST	
	LUNCH	
	DINNER	

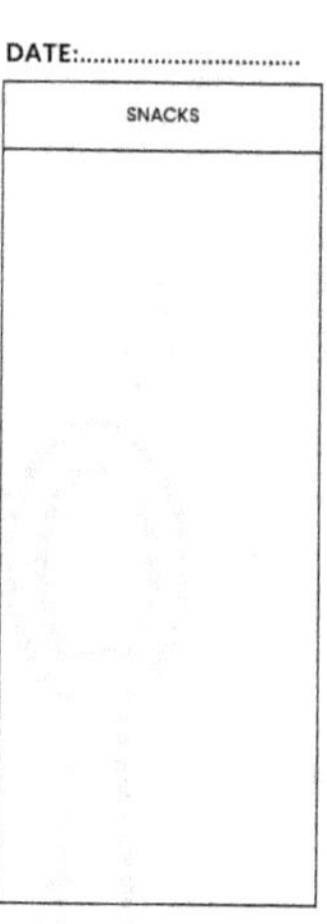

SNACKS

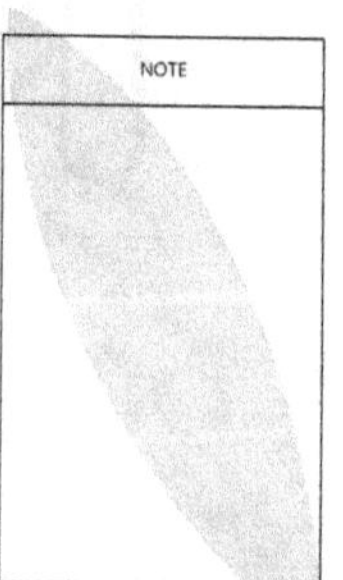

NOTE

WEEKLY MEAL JOURNAL

DATE:.................................

MONDAY	BREAKFAST	
	LUNCH	
	DINNER	
TUESDAY	BREAKFAST	
	LUNCH	
	DINNER	
WEDNESDAY	BREAKFAST	
	LUNCH	
	DINNER	
THURSDAY	BREAKFAST	
	LUNCH	
	DINNER	
FRIDAY	BREAKFAST	
	LUNCH	
	DINNER	
SATURDAY	BREAKFAST	
	LUNCH	
	DINNER	
SUNDAY	BREAKFAST	
	LUNCH	
	DINNER	

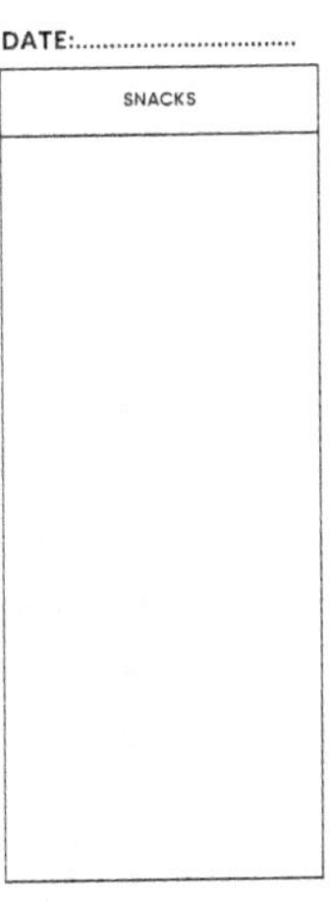

SNACKS

NOTE

WEEKLY MEAL JOURNAL

DATE:.................................

MONDAY	BREAKFAST	
	LUNCH	
	DINNER	
TUESDAY	BREAKFAST	
	LUNCH	
	DINNER	
WEDNESDAY	BREAKFAST	
	LUNCH	
	DINNER	
THURSDAY	BREAKFAST	
	LUNCH	
	DINNER	
FRIDAY	BREAKFAST	
	LUNCH	
	DINNER	
SATURDAY	BREAKFAST	
	LUNCH	
	DINNER	
SUNDAY	BREAKFAST	
	LUNCH	
	DINNER	

SNACKS

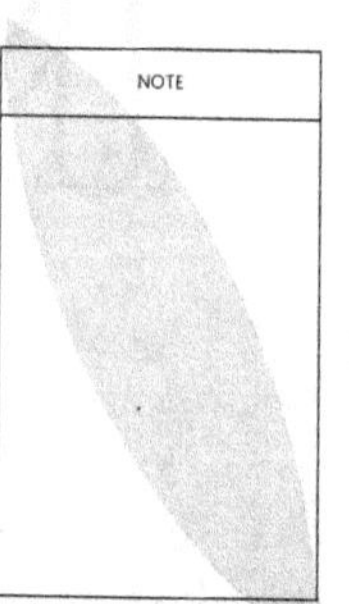

NOTE

WEEKLY MEAL JOURNAL

DATE:..................................

MONDAY	BREAKFAST	
	LUNCH	
	DINNER	
TUESDAY	BREAKFAST	
	LUNCH	
	DINNER	
WEDNESDAY	BREAKFAST	
	LUNCH	
	DINNER	
THURSDAY	BREAKFAST	
	LUNCH	
	DINNER	
FRIDAY	BREAKFAST	
	LUNCH	
	DINNER	
SATURDAY	BREAKFAST	
	LUNCH	
	DINNER	
SUNDAY	BREAKFAST	
	LUNCH	
	DINNER	

SNACKS

NOTE

WEEKLY MEAL JOURNAL

DATE:.................................

MONDAY	BREAKFAST	
	LUNCH	
	DINNER	
TUESDAY	BREAKFAST	
	LUNCH	
	DINNER	
WEDNESDAY	BREAKFAST	
	LUNCH	
	DINNER	
THURSDAY	BREAKFAST	
	LUNCH	
	DINNER	
FRIDAY	BREAKFAST	
	LUNCH	
	DINNER	
SATURDAY	BREAKFAST	
	LUNCH	
	DINNER	
SUNDAY	BREAKFAST	
	LUNCH	
	DINNER	

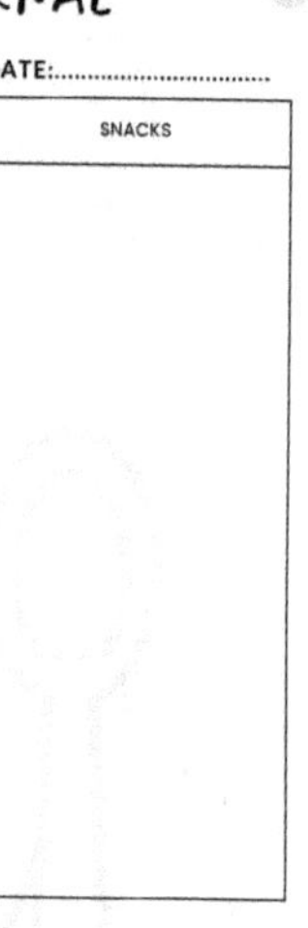

SNACKS

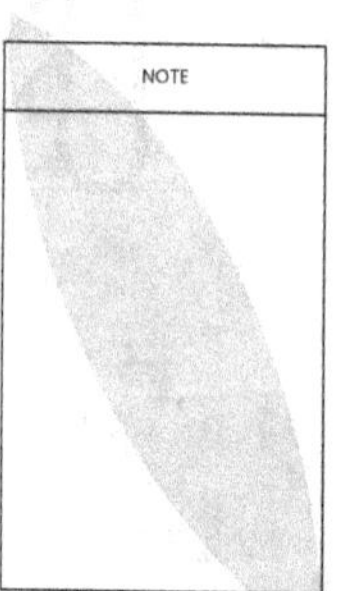

NOTE

WEEKLY MEAL JOURNAL

DATE:...................................

MONDAY	BREAKFAST	
	LUNCH	
	DINNER	
TUESDAY	BREAKFAST	
	LUNCH	
	DINNER	
WEDNESDAY	BREAKFAST	
	LUNCH	
	DINNER	
THURSDAY	BREAKFAST	
	LUNCH	
	DINNER	
FRIDAY	BREAKFAST	
	LUNCH	
	DINNER	
SATURDAY	BREAKFAST	
	LUNCH	
	DINNER	
SUNDAY	BREAKFAST	
	LUNCH	
	DINNER	

SNACKS

NOTE

WEEKLY MEAL JOURNAL

DATE:...................................

MONDAY	BREAKFAST	
	LUNCH	
	DINNER	
TUESDAY	BREAKFAST	
	LUNCH	
	DINNER	
WEDNESDAY	BREAKFAST	
	LUNCH	
	DINNER	
THURSDAY	BREAKFAST	
	LUNCH	
	DINNER	
FRIDAY	BREAKFAST	
	LUNCH	
	DINNER	
SATURDAY	BREAKFAST	
	LUNCH	
	DINNER	
SUNDAY	BREAKFAST	
	LUNCH	
	DINNER	

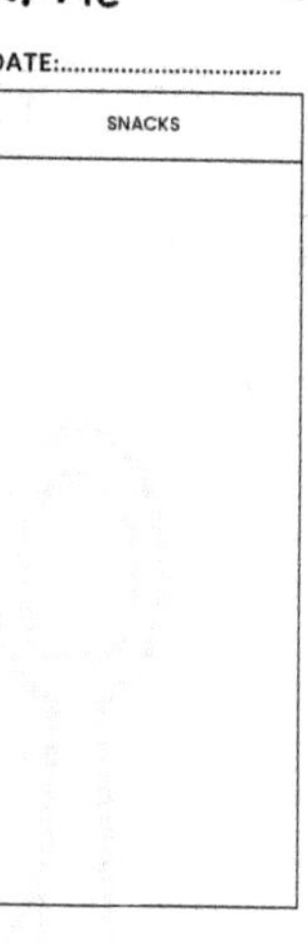

SNACKS

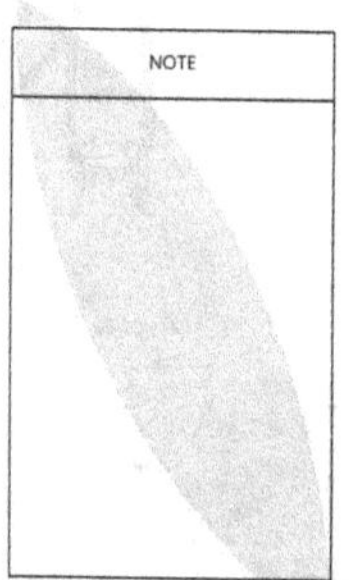

NOTE

WEEKLY MEAL JOURNAL

DATE:.................................

MONDAY	BREAKFAST	
	LUNCH	
	DINNER	
TUESDAY	BREAKFAST	
	LUNCH	
	DINNER	
WEDNESDAY	BREAKFAST	
	LUNCH	
	DINNER	
THURSDAY	BREAKFAST	
	LUNCH	
	DINNER	
FRIDAY	BREAKFAST	
	LUNCH	
	DINNER	
SATURDAY	BREAKFAST	
	LUNCH	
	DINNER	
SUNDAY	BREAKFAST	
	LUNCH	
	DINNER	

SNACKS

NOTE

WEEKLY MEAL JOURNAL

DATE:..................................

MONDAY	BREAKFAST	
	LUNCH	
	DINNER	
TUESDAY	BREAKFAST	
	LUNCH	
	DINNER	
WEDNESDAY	BREAKFAST	
	LUNCH	
	DINNER	
THURSDAY	BREAKFAST	
	LUNCH	
	DINNER	
FRIDAY	BREAKFAST	
	LUNCH	
	DINNER	
SATURDAY	BREAKFAST	
	LUNCH	
	DINNER	
SUNDAY	BREAKFAST	
	LUNCH	
	DINNER	

SNACKS

NOTE

WEEKLY MEAL JOURNAL

DATE:...................................

MONDAY	BREAKFAST	
	LUNCH	
	DINNER	
TUESDAY	BREAKFAST	
	LUNCH	
	DINNER	
WEDNESDAY	BREAKFAST	
	LUNCH	
	DINNER	
THURSDAY	BREAKFAST	
	LUNCH	
	DINNER	
FRIDAY	BREAKFAST	
	LUNCH	
	DINNER	
SATURDAY	BREAKFAST	
	LUNCH	
	DINNER	
SUNDAY	BREAKFAST	
	LUNCH	
	DINNER	

SNACKS

NOTE